The Definitive Guide to Dash Diet Meals Preparation

A Super Affordable list of Dinner Recipes to Enjoy Your Evening Meals with Taste

Maya Wilson

Table of contents

Zucchini Pasta with Pesto Sauce

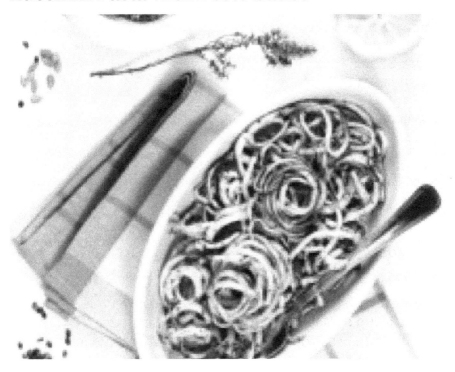

Nutritional Facts

servings per container   5
Prep Total   10 min
Serving Size 2/3 cup (20g)
Amount per serving 100
Calories

        % Daily Value
Total Fat 8g 12%
Saturated Fat 1g   2%
Trans Fat 0g 20%
Cholesterol   2%
Sodium 10mg   7%
Total Carbohydrate 7g   2%
Dietary Fiber 2g   14%

Total Sugar 1g   01.20%
Protein 3g
Vitamin C 2mcg   10%
Calcium 240mg   1%
Iron 2mg   2%
Potassium 25mg   6%

Ingredients

- 1 to 2 medium zucchini (make noodles with a mandoline or Spiralizer)
- 1/2 teaspoon of salt

For Pesto

- soaked 1/4 cup cashews
- soaked 1/4 cup pine nuts
- 1/2 cup spinach
- 1/2 cup peas you can make it fresh or frozen one
- 1/4 cup broccoli
- 1/4 cup basil leaves
- 1/2 avocado
- 1 or 2 tablespoons original olive oil
- 2 tablespoons nutritional yeast
- 1/2 teaspoon salt
- Pinch black pepper

Instructions:

1.   Place zucchini noodles in a strainer over a clean bowl

2.   Include 1/2 teaspoon of salt & let it set while preparing the pesto sauce
3.   Mix all the ingredients for the pesto sauce
4.   Extract excess water from zucchini noodles & place them in a clean bowl

5.   Pour the sauce on top & garnish with some basil leaves & pine nut

Balsamic BBQ Seitan And Tempeh Ribs

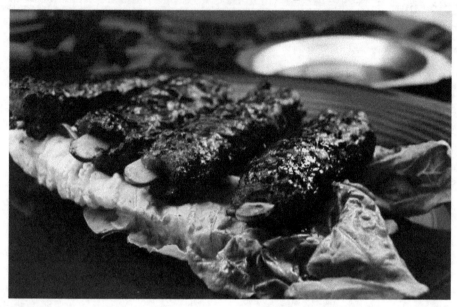

Nutritional Facts

servings per container   4
Prep Total   10 min
Serving Size 2/3 cup (56g)
Amount per serving 100
Calories

      % Daily Value
Total Fat 7g   1%
Saturated Fat 1g   2%
Trans Fat 0g 20%
Cholesterol   2%
Sodium 160mg   7%
Total Carbohydrate 37g   2%
Dietary Fiber 2g   1%
Total Sugar 2g   01.20%
Protein 14g
Vitamin C 1mcg   10%

Calcium 450mg   1%
Iron 2mg   2%
Potassium 35mg   7%

Ingredients

For the spice rub

- Minced ¼ cup fresh parsley

Instructions:

1.   In a clean bowl, join the ingredients for the spice rub. Blend well & put aside.

2.   In a small saucepan over medium heat, combine the apple juice vinegar, balsamic vinegar, maple syrup, ketchup, red onion, garlic, and chile. Mix & let stew, revealed, for around 60 minutes. Increase the level of the heat to medium-high & cook for 15 additional minutes until the sauce thickens. Mix it frequently. In the event that it appears to be excessively thick, include some water.

3.   Preheat the oven to 350 degrees. In a clean bowl, join the dry ingredients for the seitan & blend well. In a clean bowl, add the wet ingredients. Add the wet ingredients to the dry & blend until simply consolidated. Manipulate the dough gently until everything is combined & the dough feels elastic.

4.   Grease or shower a preparing dish. Include the dough to the baking dish, smoothing it & stretching it to fit the dish. Cut the dough into 7 to 9 strips & afterward down the middle to make 16 thick ribs.

5.   Top the dough with the flavor rub & back rub it in a bit. Heat the seitan for 40 minutes to an hour or until the seitan has a strong surface to it. Remove the dish from the heater. Recut the strips & cautiously remove them from the baking dish.

6.   Increase the oven temperature to about 400 degrees. Slather the ribs with BBQ sauce & lay them on a baking sheet. Set the ribs back in the heater for pretty much 12 minutes so the sauce can get a bit roasted. Then again, you can cook the sauce-covered ribs on a grill or in a grill pan.

Green Bean Casserole

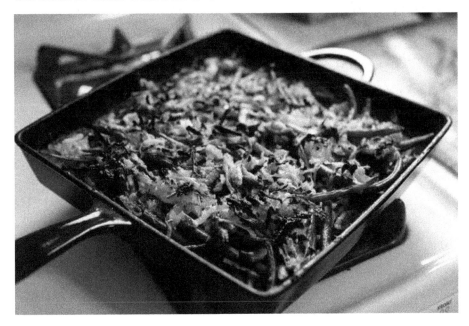

Nutritional Facts
servings per container   2

Prep Total   10 min
Serving Size 2/3 cup (5g)
Amount per serving 100
Calories

            % Daily Value
Total Fat 10g 12%
Saturated Fat 2g   2%
Trans Fat 4g 20%
Cholesterol   2%
Sodium 70mg   7%
Total Carbohydrate 18g   2%
Dietary Fiber 9g   10%
Total Sugar 16g   01.20%
Protein 2g
Vitamin C 9mcg   10%

Calcium 720mg   1%
Iron 6mg   2%
Potassium 150mg   6%

Ingredients

- Diced 1 large onion

- 3 tablespoons of original olive oil

- ¼ cup flour

- 2 cups of water

- 1 tablespoon of salt

- ½ tablespoons of garlic powder

- 1 or 2 bags frozen green beans (10 ounces each)

- 1 fried onion

Instructions:

1.   Preheat oven to 350 degrees.

2.   Heat original olive oil in a shallow pan. Include onion & stir occasionally while the onions soften and turn translucent. This takes about 15 to 20 minutes, don't rush it because it gives

so much flavor! Once onion is well cooked, include flour & stir well to cook flour. It will be a dry mixture. Include salt & garlic powder. Add some water. Let simmer for about 1 – 2 minutes & allow mixture to thicken. Immediately remove from heat

3.   Pour green beans into a square baking dish & add 2/3 can of onions. Include all of the gravy & stir well to together

4.   Place in oven & cook for 25 to 30 minutes, gravy mixture will be bubbly. Top with remaining fried onions & cook for 4 to 12 minutes more. Serve immediately and enjoy your dinner.

Socca Pizza [Vegan]

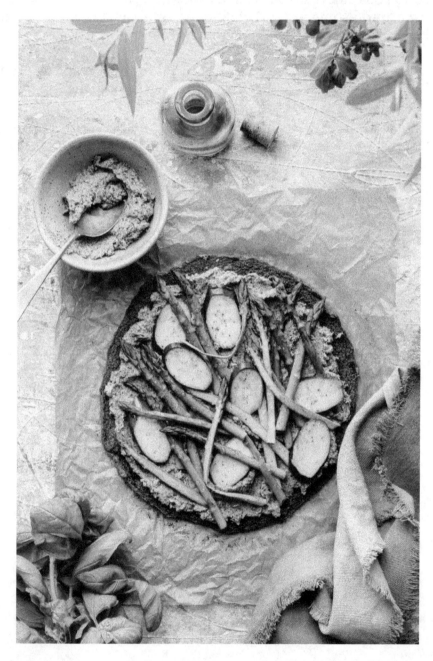

Nutritional Facts

servings per container   2
Prep Total   10 min
Serving Size 2/3 cup (78g)
Amount per serving 120
Calories

% Daily Value

Total Fat 10g	20%
Saturated Fat 5g	7%
Trans Fat 6g	27%
Cholesterol 5%	
Sodium 10mg	10%
Total Carbohydrate 4g	20%
Dietary Fiber 9g	15%
Total Sugar 12g	01.70%
Protein 6g	
Vitamin C 7mcg	10%
Calcium 290mg	20%
Iron 4mg	2%
Potassium 240mg	7%

Ingredients

- Socca Base

- 1 cup chickpea (garbanzo bean) flour – I used bob's Red Mill Garbanzo Fava Flour

- 1 or 2 cups of cold, filtered water

- 1 to 2 tablespoons minced garlic

- ½ tablespoon of sea salt

- 2 tablespoons coconut oil (for greasing)

Toppings

- Add Tomato-paste

- Add Dried Italian herbs (oregano, basil, thyme, rosemary, etc.)

- Add Mushrooms

- Add Red onion

- Add Capsicum/bell pepper

- Add Sun-dried tomatoes

- Add Kalamata olives

- Add Vegan Cheese & Chopped Fresh basil leaves

Instructions:

1. Pre-heat oven to 350F

2.   In a clean mixing bowl, whisk together garbanzo bean flour & water until there are no lumps remaining. Stir together in garlic 7 sea salt. Allow resting for about 12 minutes to thicken.

3.   Grease 2 - 4 small, shallow dishes/tins with original coconut oil

4.   Pour mixture into a clean dish & bake for about 20 - 15 minutes or until golden brown.
5.   Remove dishes from oven, top with your favorite toppings & vegan cheese (optional) & return to the oven for another 7 - 10 minutes or so.
6.   Remove dishes from oven & allow to sit for a about 2 – 5 minutes before removing pizzas from the dishes. Enjoy your dinner!

Rainbow Nourishment Bowl

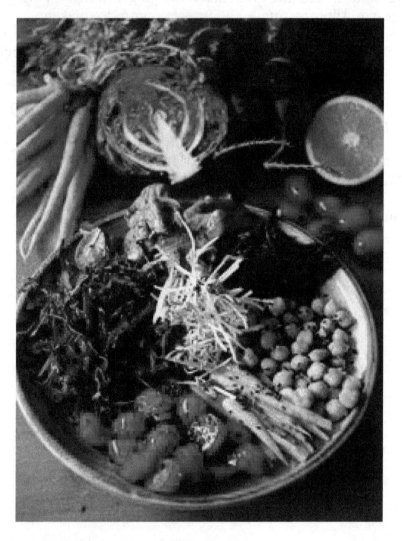

Nutritional Facts

servings per container   5
Prep Total   10 min
Serving Size 2/3 cup (77g)
Amount per serving 20
Calories

% Daily Value
Total Fat 2g   0%
Saturated Fat 7g   2%
Trans Fat 0g 10%
Cholesterol   5%

Sodium 55mg   20%
Total Carbohydrate 9g   200%
Dietary Fiber 7g   1%
Total Sugar 36g   2%
Protein 1g
Vitamin C 6mcg   21%
Calcium 160mg   2%
Iron 7mg   2%
Potassium 320mg   10%   .

Ingredients

- 2 cups spinach

- 1/2 cup corn kernels

- 1/2 cup edamame beans

- 1/2 cup cabbage, shredded

- 1/4 cup carrots, sliced

- 1/2 cup quinoa, cooked

- 1 radish, sliced

- Handful pea shoot sprouts (or another type of sprouts)

- 1/2 avocado, sliced

- Sesame seeds

- Juice of 1/2 lemon

Instructions:

1.   Start by filling the bottom of the Coconut Bowls with spinach.

2.   Place the corn, edamame, cabbage, carrots, cooked quinoa, radish, sprouts, & avocado in small piles on top of the bowls.
3.   Sprinkle with sesame seeds.
4.   Dress with some lemon juice if desired

Caramelized Banana & Blueberry Tacos

Nutritional Facts

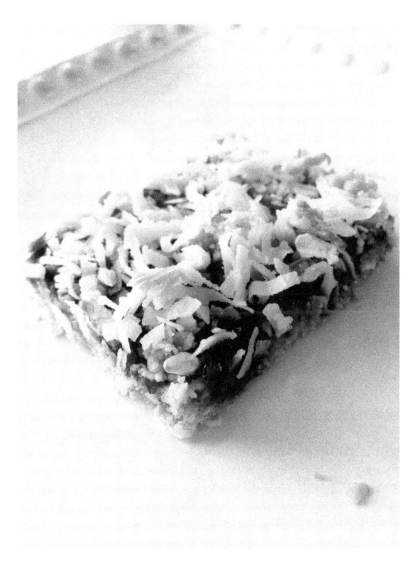

servings per container   7

Prep Total   10 min

Serving Size 2/3 cup (51g)

Amount per serving
11
Calories

% Daily Value

Total Fat 2g 2%

Saturated Fat 7g   10%

Trans Fat 3g 8%

Cholesterol   9%

Sodium 470mg   2%

Total Carbohydrate 20g   200%

Dietary Fiber 10g   20%

Total Sugar 9g   1%

Protein 6g

Vitamin C 1mcg   20%

Calcium 700mg   7%

Iron 7mg   2%

Potassium 470mg   9%

Ingredients

- 4 flour tortillas

- 1 Teaspoon coconut oil

- 2 ripe bananas, peeled and sliced lengthways into 0.5cm / 0.2" slices

- 100g / 3.5oz fresh blueberries

- 1 Teaspoon maple syrup

- 3 Teaspoon vanilla favored coconut or soy yogurt

- 1 heaped teaspoon tahini

- 1.5 Teaspoon shredded coconut or coconut flakes

- 1 Teaspoon cacao nibs

Instructions:

1.   You will need to preheat the oven to 160°C / 320°F.

2.   Kindly wrap the tortillas in foil & heat in the oven for 6 minutes.

3.   Heat a medium-sized, heavy-based, non-stick or cast-iron skillet on medium heat on the stove. Add original coconut oil & once it's melted, add the sliced clean bananas.

4.   Fry the bananas until they are golden brown on both sides, making

sure to rotate them frequently so they won't stick to the pan.

5.   You need to top the warm tortillas with the fried bananas and drizzle with tahini, yogurt, and maple syrup.

6.   Kindly top with blueberries and sprinkle with coconut and cacao nibs.

7.   Serve and enjoy

Decent Beef and Onion Stew

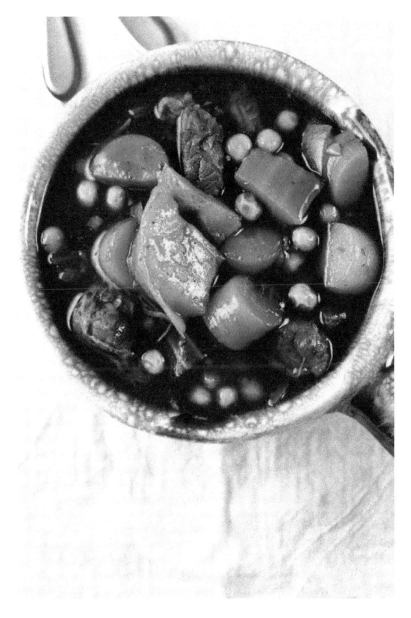

Serving: 4

Prep Time: 10 minutes

Cook Time 1-2 hours

Ingredients:

- 2 pounds lean beef, cubed

- 3 pounds shallots, peeled

- 5 garlic cloves, peeled, whole

- 3 tablespoons tomato paste

- 1 bay leaves

- ¼ cup olive oil

- 3 tablespoons lemon juice

How To:

1. Take a stew pot and place it over medium heat.
2. Add vegetable oil and let it heat up.
3. Add meat and brown.
4. Add remaining ingredients and canopy with water.
5. Bring the entire mix to a boil.
6. Reduce heat to low and canopy the pot.
7. Simmer for 1-2 hours until beef is cooked thoroughly.
8. Serve hot!

Nutrition (Per Serving)

Calories: 136

Fat: 3g

Carbohydrates: 0.9g

Protein: 24g

Clean Parsley and Chicken Breast

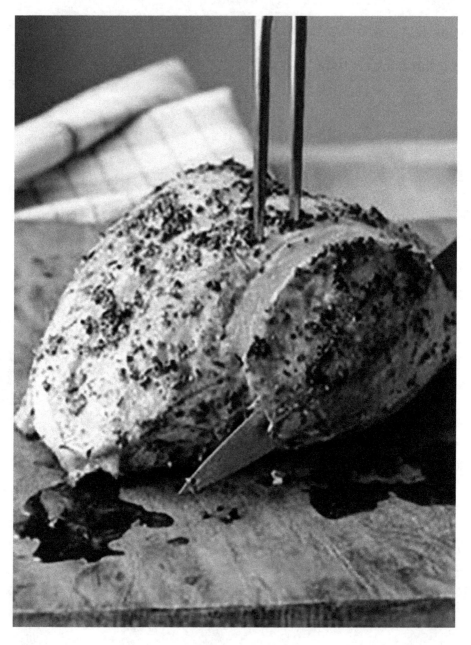

Serving: 2

Prep Time: 10 minutes

Cook Time: 40 minutes

Ingredients:

- 1/2 tablespoon dry parsley

- 1/2 tablespoon dry basil

- 2 chicken breast halves, boneless and skinless 1/4 teaspoon sunflower seeds

- 1/4 teaspoon red pepper flakes, crushed 1 tomato, sliced

How To:

1.   Pre-heat your oven to 350 degrees F.

2.   Take a 9x13 inch baking dish and grease it up with cooking spray.

3.   Sprinkle 1 tablespoon of parsley, 1 teaspoon of basil and spread the mixture over your baking dish.
4.   Arrange the pigeon breast halves over the dish and sprinkle garlic slices on top.
5.   Take a little bowl and add 1 teaspoon parsley, 1 teaspoon of basil, sunflower seeds, basil, red pepper and blend well. Pour the mixture over the pigeon breast .
6.   Top with tomato slices and canopy , bake for 25 minutes.
7.   Remove the duvet and bake for quarter-hour more.
8.   Serve and enjoy!

Nutrition (Per Serving)

Calories: 150

Fat: 4g

Carbohydrates: 4g

Protein: 25g

Zucchini Beef Sauté with Coriander Greens

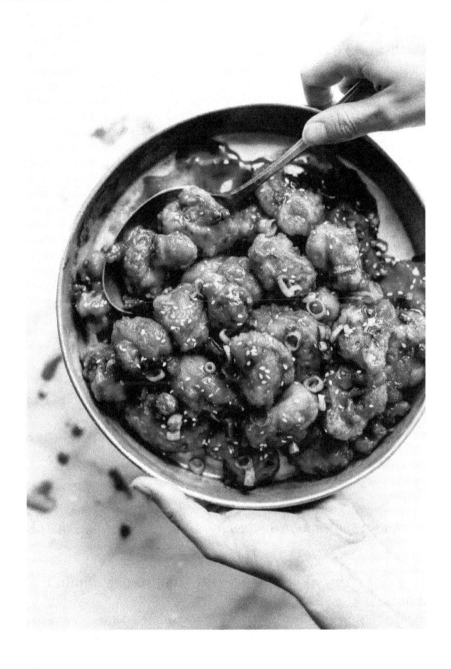

Serving: 4

Prep Time: 10 minutes

Cook Time: 10 minutes

Ingredients:

- 10 ounces beef, sliced into 1-2-inch strips

- 1 zucchini, cut into 2-inch strips

- ¼ cup parsley, chopped

- 3 garlic cloves, minced

- 2 tablespoons tamari sauce

- 4 tablespoons avocado oil

How To:

1.   Add 2 tablespoons avocado oil during a frypan over high heat.

2.   Place strips of beef and brown for a couple of minutes on high heat.

3.   Once the meat is brown, add zucchini strips and sauté until tender.

4.   Once tender, add tamari sauce, garlic, parsley and allow them to sit for a couple of minutes more.
5.   Serve immediately and enjoy!

Nutrition (Per Serving)

Calories: 500

Fat: 40g

Carbohydrates: 5g

Protein: 31g

Hearty Lemon and Pepper Chicken

Serving: 4

Prep Time: 5 minutes

Cook Time: 15

Ingredients:

- 2 teaspoons olive oil

- 1 ¼ pounds skinless chicken cutlets

- 2 whole eggs

- ¼ cup panko crumbs

- 1 tablespoon lemon pepper

- Sunflower seeds and pepper to taste

- 3 cups green beans

- ¼ cup parmesan cheese

- ¼ teaspoon garlic powder

How To:

1.   Pre-heat your oven to 425 degrees F.
2.   Take a bowl and stir in seasoning, parmesan, lemon pepper, garlic powder, panko.
3.   Whisk eggs in another bowl.
4.   Coat cutlets in eggs and press into panko mix.
5.   Transfer coated chicken to a parchment lined baking sheet.
6.   Toss the beans in oil, pepper, add sunflower seeds, and lay them on the side of the baking sheet.
7.   Bake for quarter-hour .
8.   Enjoy!

Nutrition (Per Serving)

Calorie: 299
Fat: 10g

Carbohydrates: 10g

Protein: 43g

Walnuts and Asparagus Delight

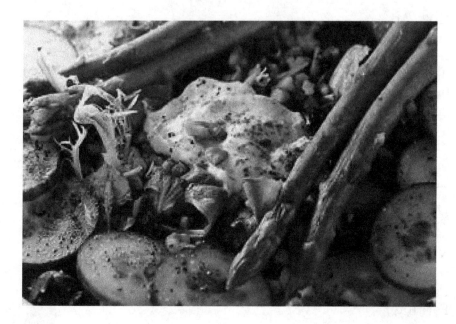

Serving: 4

Prep Time: 5 minutes

Cook Time: 5 minutes

Ingredients:

- 1 ½ tablespoons olive oil

- ¾ pound asparagus, trimmed

- ¼ cup walnuts, chopped

- Sunflower seeds and pepper to taste

How To:

1.   Place a skillet over medium heat add vegetable oil and let it heat up.
2.   Add asparagus, sauté for five minutes until browned.
3.   Season with sunflower seeds and pepper.
4.   Remove heat.
5.   Add walnuts and toss.
6.   Serve warm!

Nutrition (Per Serving)

Calories: 124

Fat: 12g

Carbohydrates: 2g

Protein: 3g

Healthy Carrot Chips

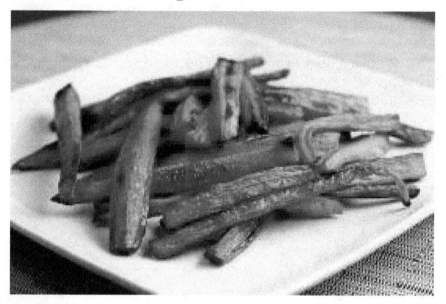

Serving: 4

Prep Time: 10 minutes

Cook Time: 10 minutes

Ingredients:

- 3 cups carrots, sliced paper-thin rounds

- 2 tablespoons olive oil

- 2 teaspoons ground cumin

- ½ teaspoon smoked paprika Pinch of sunflower seeds

How To:

1.   Pre-heat your oven to 400 degrees F.

2.   Slice carrot into thin shaped coins employing a peeler.
3.   Place slices during a bowl and toss with oil and spices.
4.   Lay out the slices on a parchment paper, lined baking sheet during a single layer.

5.   Sprinkle sunflower seeds.

6.   Transfer to oven and bake for 8-10 minutes.
7.   Remove and serve.

Enjoy!

Nutrition (Per Serving)

Calories: 434

Fat: 35g

Carbohydrates: 31g

Protein: 2g

Beef Soup

Serving: 4

Prep Time: 10 minutes

Cook Time: 40 minutes

Ingredients:

- 1-pound ground beef, lean

- 1 cup mixed vegetables, frozen

- 1 yellow onion, chopped

- 6 cups vegetable broth

- 1 cup low-fat cream Pepper to taste

How To: ,

1.   Take a stockpot and add all the ingredients the except cream , salt, and black pepper.

2.   bring back a boil.
3.   Reduce heat to simmer.
4.   Cook for 40 minutes.
5.   Once cooked, warm the cream .
6.   Then add once the soup is cooked.
7.   Blend the soup till smooth by using an immersion blender.
8.   Season with salt and black pepper.

9.   Serve and enjoy!

Nutrition (Per Serving)

Calories: 270

Fat: 14g

Carbohydrates: 6g

Protein: 29g

Amazing Grilled Chicken and Blueberry Salad

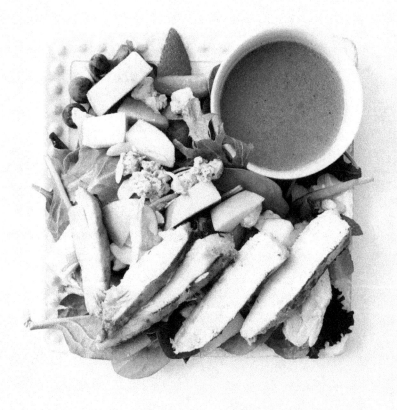

Serving: 5

Prep Time: 10 minutes

Cook Time: 25 minutes

Smart Points: 9

Ingredients:

- 5 cups mixed greens

- 1 cup blueberries

- ¼ cup slivered almonds

- 2 cups chicken breasts, cooked and cubed

- For dressing

- ¼ cup olive oil

- ¼ cup apple cider vinegar

- ¼ cup blueberries

- 2 tablespoons honey

- Sunflower seeds and pepper to taste

How To:

1.   Take a bowl and add greens, berries, almonds, chicken cubes and blend well.

2.   Take a bowl and blend the dressing ingredients, pour the combination into a blender and blitz until smooth.
3.   Add dressing on top of the chicken cubes and toss well.
4.   Season more and enjoy!

Nutrition (Per Serving)

Calories: 266

Fat: 17g

Carbohydrates: 18g

Protein: 10g

Clean Chicken and Mushroom Stew

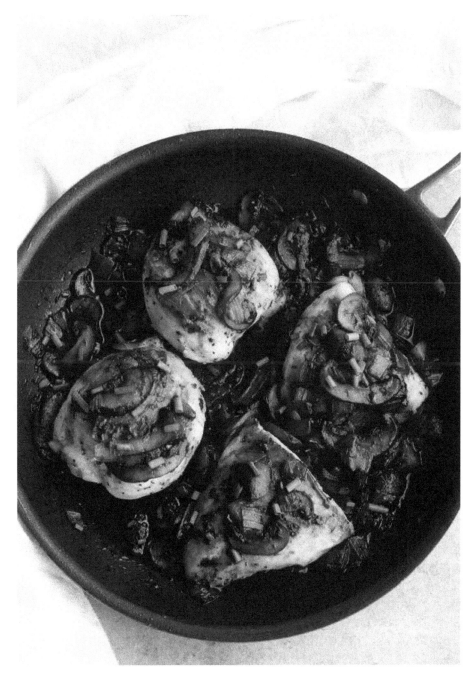

Serving: 4

Prep Time: 10 minutes

Cook Time: 35 minutes

Ingredients:

- 4 chicken breast halves, cut into bite sized pieces

- 1 pound mushrooms, sliced (5-6 cups)

- 1 bunch spring onion, chopped

- 4 tablespoons olive oil

- 1 teaspoon thyme

- Sunflower seeds and pepper as needed

How To:

1.   Take an outsized deep frypan and place it over medium-high heat.
2.   Add oil and let it heat up.
3.   Add chicken and cook for 4-5 minutes per side until slightly browned.
4.   Add spring onions and mushrooms, season with sunflower seeds and pepper consistent with your taste.

5.   Stir.
6.   Cover with lid and convey the combination to a boil.
7.   Reduce heat and simmer for 25 minutcs.
8.   Serve!

Nutrition (Per Serving)

Calories: 247

Fat: 12g

Carbohydrates: 10g

Protein: 23g

Elegant Pumpkin Chili Dish

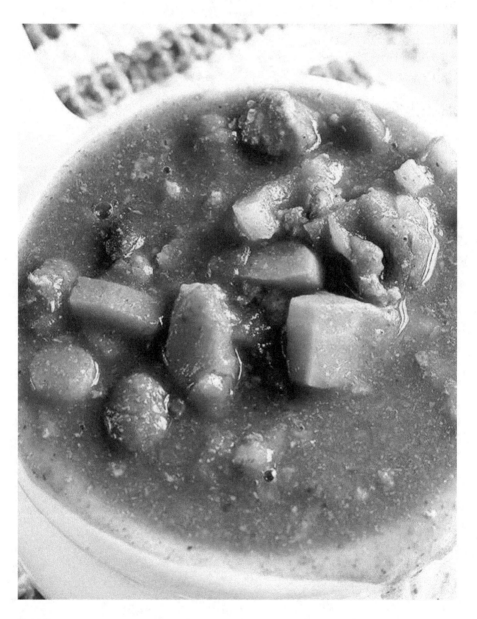

Serving: 4

Prep Time: 10 minutes

Cook Time: 15 minutes

Ingredients:

- 3 cups yellow onion, chopped

- 8 garlic cloves, chopped

- 1 pound turkey, ground

- 2 cans (15 ounces each) fire roasted tomatoes

- 2 cups pumpkin puree

- 1 cup chicken broth

- 4 teaspoons chili spice

- 1 teaspoon ground cinnamon

- 1 teaspoon sea sunflower seeds

How To:

1.	Take an outsized sized pot and place it over medium-high heat.

2.	Add copra oil and let the oil heat up.
3.	Add onion and garlic, sauté for five minutes.
4.	Add ground turkey and break it while cooking, cook for five minutes.
5.	Add remaining ingredients and convey the combination to simmer.

6.	Simmer for quarter-hour over low heat (lid off).
7.	Pour chicken stock .
8.	Serve with desired salad.
9.	Enjoy!

Nutrition (Per Serving)

Calories: 312

Fat: 16g

Carbohydrates: 14g

Protein: 27g

Zucchini Zoodles with Chicken and Basil

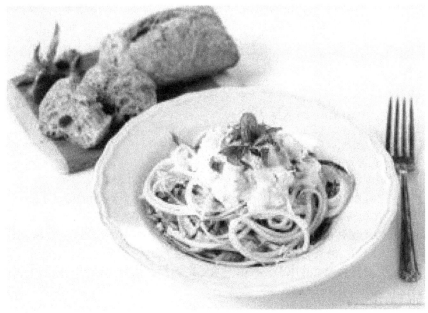

Serving: 2

Prep Time: 10 minutes

Cook Time: 10 minutes

Ingredients:

- 2 chicken fillets, cubed

- 2 tablespoons ghee

- 1-pound tomatoes, diced

- ½ cup basil, chopped

- ¼ cup coconut almond milk

- 1 garlic clove, peeled, minced

- 1 zucchini, shredded

How To:

1.   Sauté cubed chicken in ghee until not pink.
2.   Add tomatoes and season with sunflower seeds.
3.   Simmer and reduce the liquid.
4.   Prepare your zucchini Zoodles by shredding zucchini during a kitchen appliance .
5.   Add basil, garlic, coconut almond milk to chicken and cook for a couple of minutes.
6.   Add half the zucchini Zoodles to a bowl and top with creamy tomato basil chicken.
7.   Enjoy!

Nutrition (Per Serving)

Calories: 540

Fat: 27g

Carbohydrates: 13g

Protein: 59g

Tasty Roasted Broccoli

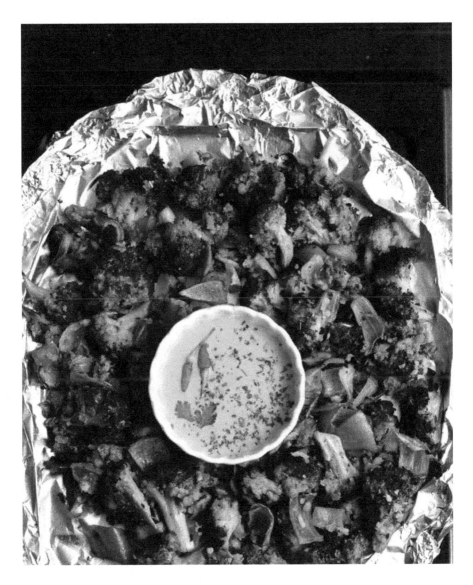

Serving: 4

Prep Time: 5 minutes

Cook Time: 20 minutes

Ingredients:

- 4 cups broccoli florets

- 1 tablespoon olive oil

- Sunflower seeds and pepper to taste

How To:

1. Pre-heat your oven to 400 degrees F.

2. Add broccoli during a zip bag alongside oil and shake until coated.

3. Add seasoning and shake again.
4. Spread broccoli out on baking sheet, bake for 20 minutes.
5. Let it cool and serve.
6. Enjoy!

Nutrition (Per Serving)

Calories: 62

Fat: 4g

Carbohydrates: 4g

Protein: 4g

The Almond Breaded Chicken Goodness

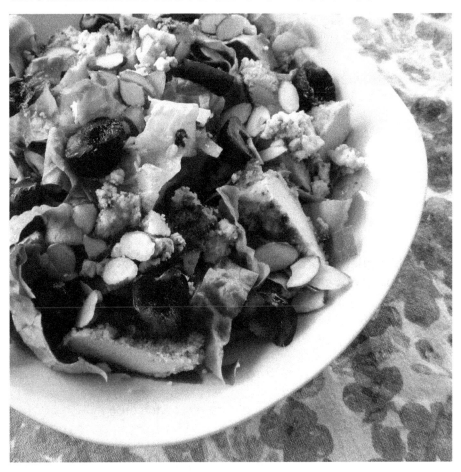

Serving: 3

Prep Time: 15 minutes

Cook Time: 15 minutes

Ingredients:

- 2 large chicken breasts, boneless and skinless 1/3 cup lemon juice

- 1 ½ cups seasoned almond meal

- 2 tablespoons coconut oil

- Lemon pepper, to taste

- Parsley for decoration

How To:
1.   Slice pigeon breast in half.
2.   Pound out each half until ¼ inch thick.
3.   Take a pan and place it over medium heat, add oil and warmth it up.
4.   Dip each pigeon breast slice through juice and let it sit for two minutes.
5.   Turnover and therefore the let the opposite side sit for two minutes also .
6.   Transfer to almond meal and coat each side .
7.   Add coated chicken to the oil and fry for 4 minutes per side, ensuring to sprinkle lemon pepper liberally.
8.   Transfer to a paper lined sheet and repeat until all chicken are fried.
9.   Garnish with parsley and enjoy!

Nutrition (Per Serving)

Calories: 325

Fat: 24g

Carbohydrates: 3g

Protein: 16g

South-Western Pork Chops

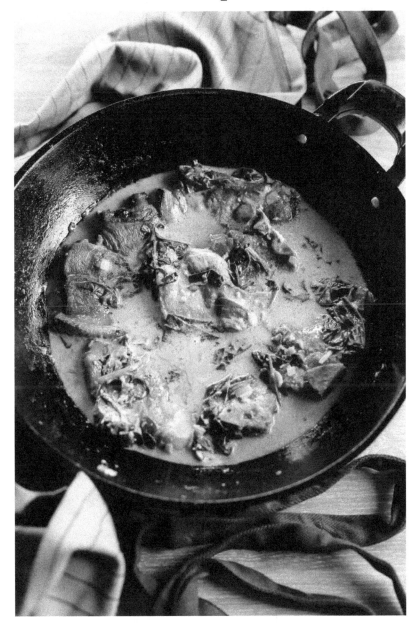

Serving: 4

Prep Time: 10 minutes

Cook Time: 15 minutes

Smart Points: 3

Ingredients:

- Cooking spray as needed 4-ounce pork loin chop, boneless and fat rimmed 1/3 cup salsa

- 2 tablespoons fresh lime juice

- ¼ cup fresh cilantro, chopped

How To:

1. Take an outsized sized non-stick skillet and spray it with cooking spray.

2. Heat until hot over high heat.
3. Press the chops together with your palm to flatten them slightly.

4. Add them to the skillet and cook on 1 minute for every side until they're nicely browned.
5. Lower the warmth to medium-low.
6. Combine the salsa and juice .
7. Pour the combination over the chops.
8. Simmer uncovered for about 8 minutes until the chops are perfectly done.
9. If needed, sprinkle some cilantro on top.
10. Serve!

Nutrition (Per Serving)

Calorie: 184
Fat: 4g
Carbohydrates: 4g
Protein: 0.5g

Almond butter Pork Chops

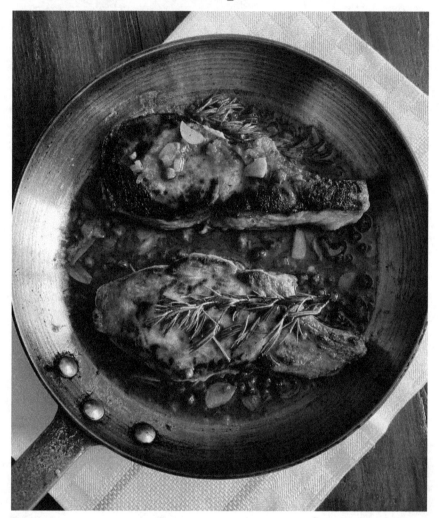

Serving: 2

Prep Time: 5 minutes

Cook Time: 25 minutes

Ingredients:

- 1 tablespoon almond butter, divided

- 2 boneless pork chops

- Pepper to taste

- 1 tablespoon dried Italian seasoning, low fat and low sodium

- 1 tablespoon olive oil

How To:
1.   Pre-heat your oven to 350 degrees F.
2.   Pat pork chops dry with a towel and place them during a baking dish.
3.   Season with pepper, and Italian seasoning.
4.   Drizzle vegetable oil over pork chops.
5.   Top each chop with ½ tablespoon almond butter.
6.   Bake for 25 minutes.
7.   Transfer pork chops on two plates and top with almond butter juice.
8.   Serve and enjoy!

Nutrition (Per Serving)

Calories: 333
Fat: 23g
Carbohydrates: 1g
Protein: 31g

Chicken Salsa

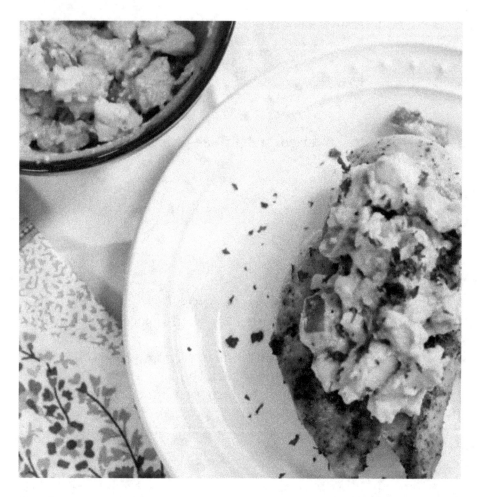

Serving: 1

Prep Time: 4 minutes

Cook Time: 14 minutes

Ingredients:

- 2 chicken breasts

- 1 cup salsa

- 1 taco seasoning mix

- 1 cup plain Greek Yogurt

- ½ cup of kite ricottta/cashew cheese, cubed

How To:

1.   Take a skillet and place over medium heat.

2.   Add pigeon breast , ½ cup of salsa and taco seasoning.
3.   Mix well and cook for 12-15 minutes until the chicken is completed .
4.   Take the back off and cube them.
5.   Place the cubes on toothpick and top with cheddar.
6.   Place yogurt and remaining salsa in cups and use as dips.

7. Enjoy!

Nutrition (Per Serving)
Calories: 359
Fat: 14g
Net Carbohydrates: 14g
Protein: 43g

Healthy Mediterranean Lamb Chops

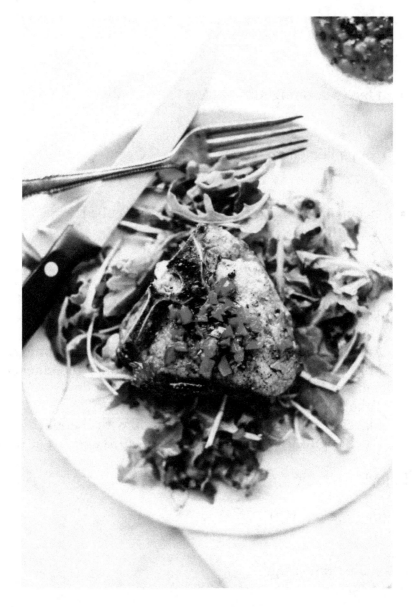

Serving: 4

Prep Time: 10 minutes

Amazing Sesame Breadsticks

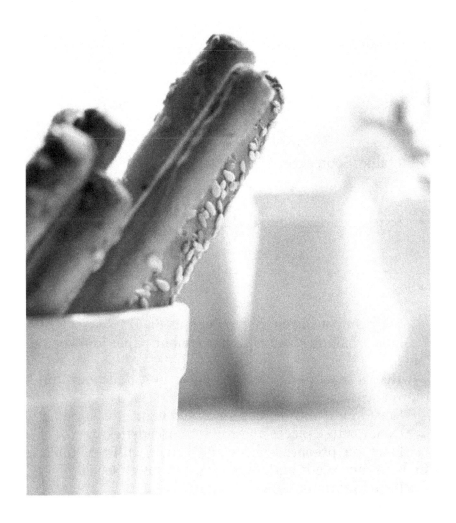

Serving: 5 breadsticks

Prep Time: 10 minutes

Cooking Time: 20 minutes

Ingredients:

- 1 egg white

- 2 tablespoons almond flour

- 1 teaspoon Himalayan pink sunflower seeds

- 1 tablespoon extra-virgin olive oil

- ½ teaspoon sesame seeds

How To:

1. Pre-heat your oven to 320 degrees F.
2. Line a baking sheet with parchment paper and keep it on the side.
3. Take a bowl and whisk in egg whites, add flour and half sunflower seeds and vegetable oil .
4. Knead until you've got a smooth dough.
5. Divide into 4 pieces and roll into breadsticks.
6. Place on prepared sheet and brush with vegetable oil , sprinkle sesame seeds and remaining sunflower seeds.
7. Bake for 20 minutes.
8. Serve and enjoy!

Nutrition (Per Serving)

Total Carbs: 1.1g
Fiber: 1g
Protein: 1.6g
Fat: 5g

Brown Butter Duck Breast

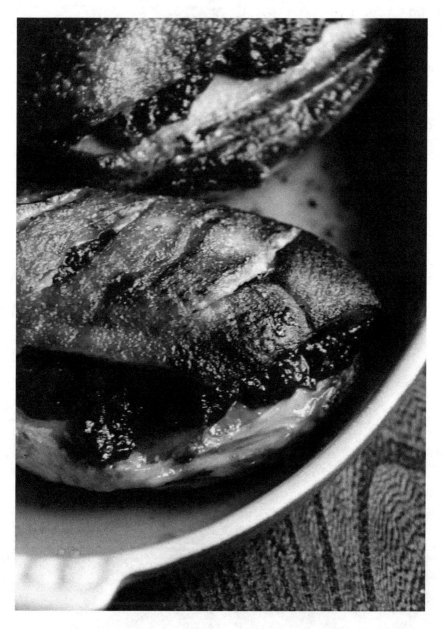

Serving: 3

Prep Time: 5 minutes

Cook Time: 25 minutes

Ingredients:

- 1 whole 6 ounce duck breast, skin on

- Pepper to taste

- 1 head radicchio, 4 ounces, core removed ¼ cup unsalted butter

- 6 fresh sage leaves, sliced

How To:

1.   Pre-heat your oven to 400 degree F.

2.   Pat duck breast dry with towel .
3.   Season with pepper.
4.   Place duck breast in skillet and place it over medium heat, sear for 3-4 minutes all sides
5.   Turn breast over and transfer skillet to oven.
6.   Roast for 10 minutes (uncovered).
7.   Cut radicchio in half.
8.   Remove and discard the woody white core and thinly slice the leaves.
9.   Keep them on the side.
10.   Remove skillet from oven.
11.   Transfer duck breast, fat side up to chopping board and let it rest.12.   Re-heat your skillet over medium heat.

13. Add unsalted butter, sage and cook for 3-4 minutes.
14.   Cut duck into 6 equal slices.
15.   Divide radicchio between 2 plates, top with slices of duck breast and drizzle browned butter and sage.
16.   Enjoy!

Nutrition (Per Serving)

Calories: 393

Fat: 33g

Carbohydrates: 2g

Protein: 22g

Generous Garlic Bread Stick

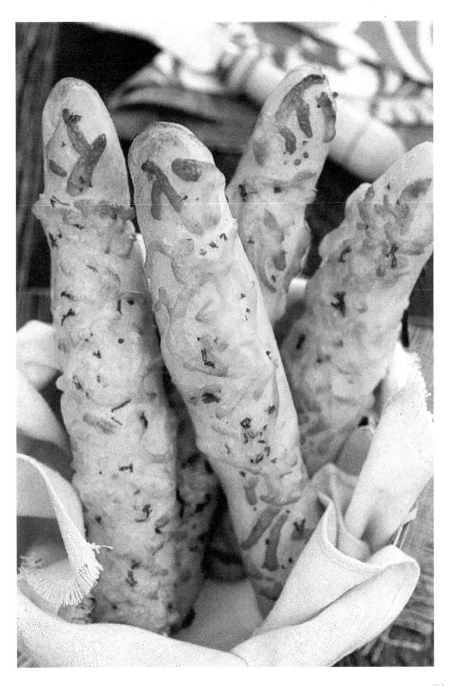

Serving: 8 breadsticks

Prep Time: 15 minutes

Cooking Time: 15 minutes

Ingredients:

- ¼ cup almond butter, softened

- 1 teaspoon garlic powder

- 2 cups almond flour

- ½ tablespoon baking powder

- 1 tablespoon Psyllium husk powder

- ¼ teaspoon sunflower seeds

- 3 tablespoons almond butter, melted
- 1 egg

- ¼ cup boiling water

How To:

1.   Pre-heat your oven to 400 degrees F.

2.   Line baking sheet with parchment paper and keep it on the side.

3.   Beat almond butter with garlic powder and keep it on the side.

4.   Add almond flour, leaven , husk, sunflower seeds during a bowl and blend in almond butter and egg, mix well.

5.   Pour boiling water within the mix and stir until you've got a pleasant dough.

6.   Divide the dough into 8 balls and roll into breadsticks.
7.   Place on baking sheet and bake for quarter-hour .
8.   Brush each persist with garlic almond butter and bake for five minutes more.
9.   Serve and enjoy!

Nutrition (Per Serving)

Total Carbs: 7g

Fiber: 2g

Protein: 7g

Fat: 24g

Cauliflower Bread Stick

Serving: 5 breadsticks

Prep Time: 10 minutes

Cooking Time: 48 minutes

Ingredients:

- 1 cup cashew cheese/ kite ricotta cheese

- 1 tablespoon organic almond butter

- 1 whole egg

- ½ teaspoon Italian seasoning

- ¼ teaspoon red pepper flakes

- 1/8 teaspoon kosher sunflower seeds

- 2 ups cauliflower rice, cooked for 3 minutes in microwave
- 3 teaspoons garlic, minced

- Parmesan cheese, grated

How To:

1.   Pre-heat your oven to 350 degrees F.

2.   Add almond butter during a small pan and melt over low heat

3.   Add red pepper flakes, garlic to the almond butter and cook for 2-3 minutes.

4.   Add garlic and almond butter mix to the bowl with cooked cauliflower and add the Italian seasoning.

5.   Season with sunflower seeds and blend , refrigerate for 10 minutes.

6.   Add cheese and eggs to the bowl and blend .

7.   Place a layer of parchment paper at rock bottom of a 9 x 9 baking dish and grease with cooking spray, add egg and mozzarella cheese mix to the cauliflower mix.

8.   Add mix to the pan and smooth to a skinny layer with the palms of your hand.

9.   Bake for half-hour , remove from oven and top with few shakes of parmesan and mozzarella.

10.   Cook for 8 minutes more.

11.   Enjoy!

Nutrition (Per Serving)

Total Carbs: 11.5g

Fiber: 2g

Protein: 10.7g

Fat: 20g

Bacon and Chicken Garlic Wrap

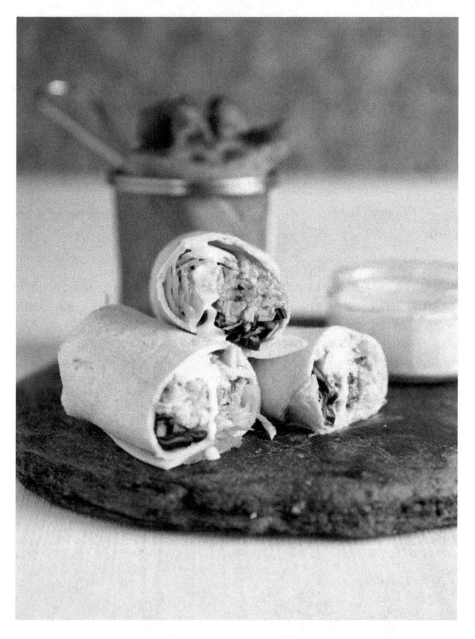

Serving: 4

Chipotle Lettuce Chicken

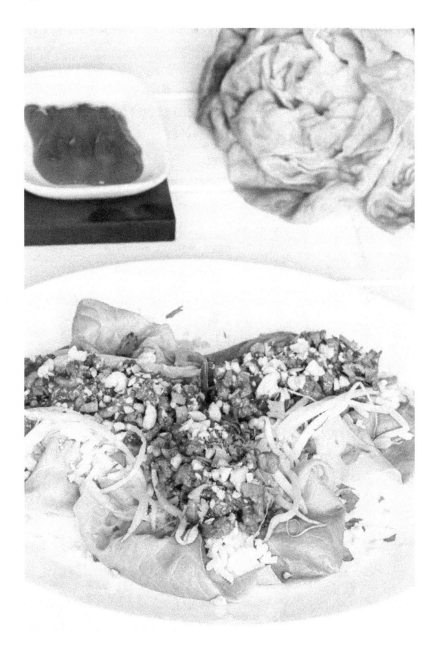

Serving: 6

Prep Time: 10 minutes

Cook Time: 25 minutes

Ingredients:

- 1-pound chicken breast, cut into strips

- Splash of olive oil

- 1 red onion, finely sliced

- 14 ounces tomatoes

- 1 teaspoon chipotle, chopped

- ½ teaspoon cumin

- Lettuce as needed

- Fresh coriander leaves

- Jalapeno chilies, sliced

- Fresh tomato slices for garnish

- Lime wedges

How To:

1. Take a non-stick frypan and place it over medium heat.

2. Add oil and warmth it up.
3. Add chicken and cook until brown.
4. Keep the chicken on the side.

5. Add tomatoes, sugar, chipotle, cumin to an equivalent pan and simmer for 25 minutes until you've got a pleasant sauce.

6. Add chicken into the sauce and cook for five minutes.
7. Transfer the combination to a different place.
8. Use lettuce wraps to require some of the mixture and serve with a squeeze of lemon.
9. Enjoy!

Nutrition (Per Serving)

Calories: 332

Fat: 15g

Carbohydrates: 13g

Protein: 34g

Balsamic Chicken and Vegetables

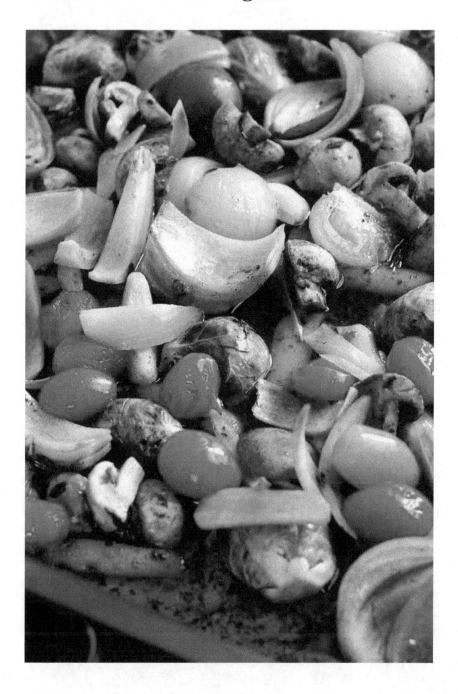

Serving: 2

Prep Time: 15 minutes

Cook Time: 25 minutes

Ingredients:

- 4 chicken thigh, boneless and skinless

- 5 stalks of asparagus, halved

- 1 pepper, cut in chunks

- 1/2 red onion, diced

- ½ cup carrots, sliced

- 1 garlic cloves, minced

- 2-ounces mushrooms, diced

- ¼ cup balsamic vinegar

- 1 tablespoon olive oil

- ½ teaspoon stevia

- ½ tablespoon oregano

- Sunflower seeds and pepper as needed

How To:

1. Pre-heat your oven to 425 degrees F.

2.   Take a bowl and add all of the vegetables and blend .

3.   Add spices and oil and blend .
4.   Dip the chicken pieces into spice mix and coat them well.
5.   Place the veggies and chicken onto a pan during a single layer.

6.   Cook for 25 minutes.
7.   Serve and enjoy!

Nutrition (Per Serving)

Calories: 401

Fat: 17g

Net Carbohydrates: 11g

Protein: 48g

Cream Dredged Corn Platter

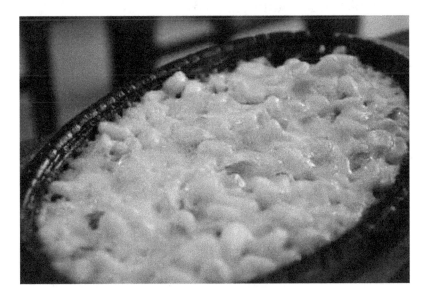

Serving: 3

Prep Time: 10 minutes

Cook Time: 4 hours

Ingredients:

- 3 cups corn

- 2 ounces cream cheese, cubed

- 2 tablespoons milk

- 2 tablespoons whipping cream

- 2 tablespoons butter, melted

- Salt and pepper as needed

- 1 tablespoon green onion, chopped

How To:

1.   Add corn, cheese , milk, light whipping cream , butter, salt and pepper to your Slow Cooker.

2.   provides it a pleasant toss to combine everything well.
3.   Place lid and cook on LOW for 4 hours.
4.   Divide the combination amongst serving platters.
5.   Serve and enjoy!

Nutrition (Per Serving)

Calories: 261

Fat: 11g

Carbohydrates: 17g

Protein: 6g

Exuberant Sweet Potatoes

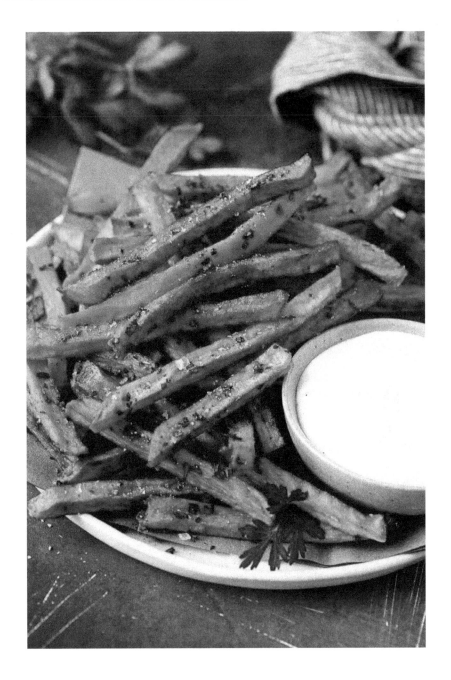

Serving: 4

Prep Time: 5 minutes

Cook Time: 7-8 hours

Ingredients:

- 6 sweet potatoes, washed and dried

How To:

1.   Loosely botch 7-8 pieces of aluminium foil within the bottom of your Slow Cooker, covering about half the area .

2.   Prick each potato 6-8 times employing a fork.
3.   Wrap each potato with foil and seal them.
4.   Place wrapped potatoes within the cooker on top of the foil bed.

5.   Place lid and cook on LOW for 7-8 hours.
6.   Use tongs to get rid of the potatoes and unwrap them.
7.   Serve and enjoy!

Nutrition (Per Serving)

Calories: 129

Fat: 0g

Carbohydrates: 30g

Protein: 2g

Ethiopian Cabbage Delight

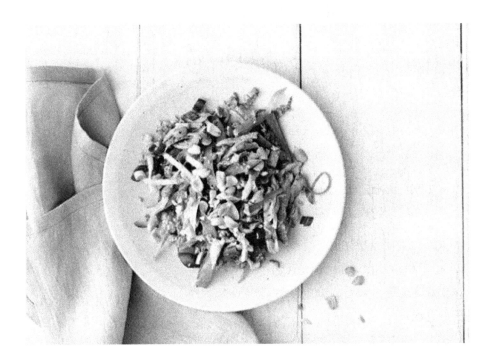

Serving: 6

Prep Time: 15 minutes

Cook Time: 6- 8 hours

Ingredients:

- ½ cup water

- 1 head green cabbage, cored and chopped

- 1-pound sweet potatoes, peeled and chopped

- 3 carrots, peeled and chopped

- 1 onion, sliced

- 1 teaspoon extra virgin olive oil

- ½ teaspoon ground turmeric
- ½ teaspoon ground cumin

- ¼ teaspoon ground ginger

How To:

1.   Add water to your Slow Cooker.
2.   Take a medium bowl and add cabbage, carrots, sweet potatoes, onion and blend .
3.   Add vegetable oil , turmeric, ginger, cumin and toss until the veggies are fully coated.
4.   Transfer veggie mix to your Slow Cooker.
5.   Cover and cook on LOW for 6-8 hours.
6.   Serve and enjoy!

Nutrition (Per Serving)

Calories: 155

Fat: 2g

Carbohydrates: 35g

Protein: 4g

Spice Trade Beans and Bulgur

Total Time

Prep: 30 min. Cook: 3-1/2 hours

Makes

10 servings

Ingredients:

- 3 tablespoons canola oil, isolated

- 2 medium onions, slashed

- 1 medium sweet red pepper, slashed

- 5 garlic cloves, minced

- 1 tablespoon ground cumin

- 1 tablespoon paprika

- 2 teaspoons ground ginger

- 1 teaspoon pepper

- 1/2 teaspoon ground cinnamon

- 1/2 teaspoon cayenne pepper

- 1-1/2 cups bulgur

- 1 can (28 ounces) squashed tomatoes

- 1 can (14-1/2 ounces) diced tomatoes, undrained

- 1 container (32 ounces) vegetable juices

- 2 tablespoons darker sugar

- 2 tablespoons soy sauce

- 1 can (15 ounces) garbanzo beans or chickpeas, flushed and depleted

- 1/2 cup brilliant raisins

- Minced crisp cilantro, discretionary

Directions:

1.   In an enormous skillet, heat 2 tablespoons oil over medium-high warmth. Include onions and pepper; cook and mix until delicate, 3-4 minutes. Include garlic and seasonings; cook brief longer. Move to a 5-qt. slow cooker.

2.   In the same skillet, heat remaining oil over medium-high warmth. Include bulgur; cook and mix until daintily caramelized, 2-3 minutes or until softly sautéed.
3.   Include bulgur, tomatoes, stock, darker sugar, and soy sauce to slow cooker. Cook, secured, on low 3-4 hours or until bulgur is

delicate. Mix in beans and raisins; cook 30 minutes longer.

Whenever wanted, sprinkle with cilantro.

Tofu Chow Mein

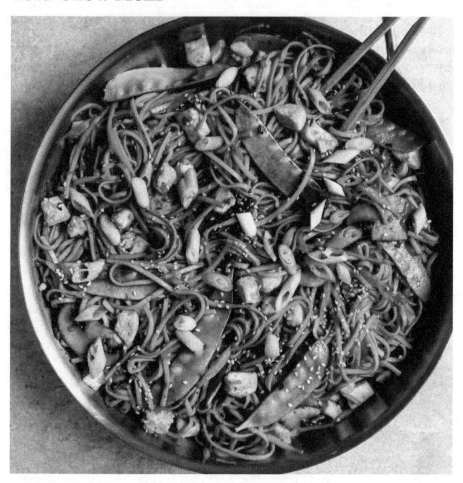

Total Time

Prep: 15 min. + standing Cook: 15 min.

Makes

4 servings

Ingredients:

- 8 ounces uncooked entire wheat holy messenger hair pasta

- 3 tablespoons sesame oil, separated

- 1 bundle (16 ounces) extra-firm tofu

- 2 cups cut new mushrooms

- 1 medium sweet red pepper, julienned

- 1/4 cup decreased sodium soy sauce

- 3 green onions daintily cut

Directions:

1.   Cook pasta as per bundle headings. Channel; flush with cold water and channel once more. Hurl with 1 tablespoon oil; spread onto a preparing sheet and let remain around 60 minutes.

2.   In the meantime, cut tofu into 1/2-in. 3D shapes and smudge dry. Enclose by a spotless kitchen towel; place on a plate and refrigerate until prepared to cook.

3.   In an enormous skillet, heat 1 tablespoon oil over medium warmth. Include pasta, spreading equitably; cook until base is daintily caramelized, around 5 minutes. Expel from skillet.

4.   In the same skillet, heat remaining oil over medium-high warmth; pan sear mushrooms, pepper, and tofu until mushrooms

are delicate, 3-4 minutes. Include pasta and soy sauce; hurl and warmth through. Sprinkle with green onions.

Salad Chard and White Bean Pasta

Total Time

Prep: 20 min. Cook: 20 min.

Makes

8 servings

Ingredients:

- 1 bundle (12 ounces) uncooked entire wheat or darker rice penne pasta

- 2 tablespoons olive oil

- 4 cups cut leeks (a white bit as it were)

- 1 cup cut sweet onion

- 4 garlic cloves, cut

- 1 tablespoon minced crisp savvy or 1 teaspoon scoured sage

- 1 enormous sweet potato, stripped and cut into 1/2-inch solid shapes

- 1 medium bundle Swiss chard (around 1 pound), cut into 1-inch cuts

- 1 can (15-1/2 ounces) extraordinary northern beans, flushed and depleted

- 3/4 teaspoon salt

- 1/4 teaspoon bean stew powder

- 1/4 teaspoon squashed red pepper drops 1/8 teaspoon ground nutmeg 1/8 teaspoon pepper

- 1/3 cup finely slashed crisp basil

- 1 tablespoon balsamic vinegar

- 2 cups marinara sauce, warmed

Directions:

1.   Cook pasta as indicated by bundle headings. Channel, holding 3/4 cup pasta water.

2.   In a 6-qt. stockpot, heat oil over medium warmth; saute leeks and onion until delicate, 5-7 minutes. Include garlic and sage; cook and mix 2 minutes.

3.   Include potato and chard; cook, secured, over medium-low warmth 5 minutes. Mix in beans, seasonings and held pasta water; cook, secured, until potato and chard are delicate, around 5 minutes.

4.   Include pasta, basil, and vinegar; hurl and warmth through. Present with sauce.

Cauliflower with Roasted Almond and Pepper Dip

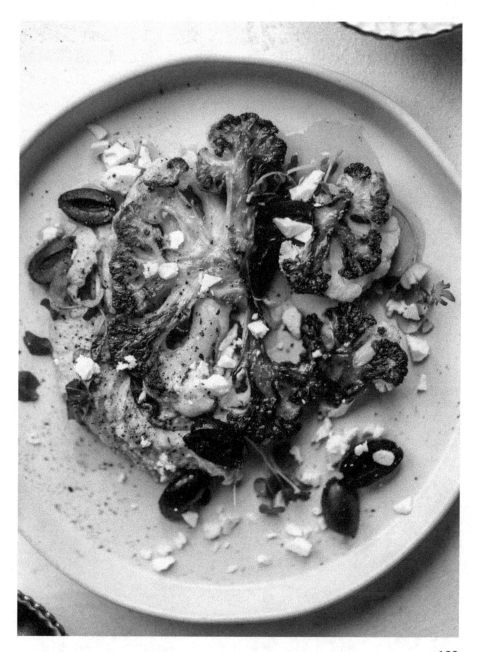

Ingredients:

Total Time

Prep: 40 min. Bake: 35 min.

Makes

10 servings (2-1/4 cups dip)

Ingredients:

- 10 cups water

- 1 cup olive oil, isolated

- 3/4 cup sherry or red wine vinegar, isolated

- 3 tablespoons salt

- 1 cove leaf

- 1 tablespoon squashed red pepper drops

- 1 enormous head cauliflower

- 1/2 cup entire almonds, toasted

- 1/2 cup delicate entire wheat or white bread morsels, toasted 1/2 cup fire-simmered squashed tomatoes

- 1 container (8 ounces) broiled sweet red peppers, depleted

- 2 tablespoons minced new parsley

- 2 garlic cloves

- 1 teaspoon sweet paprika

- 1/2 teaspoon salt

- 1/4 teaspoon newly ground pepper

Directions:

1.   In a 6-qt. stockpot, bring water, 1/2 cup oil, 1/2 cup sherry, salt, sound leaf, and pepper pieces to a bubble. Include cauliflower. Diminish heat; stew, revealed, until a blade effectively embeds into focus, 15-20 minutes, turning part of the way through cooking. Evacuate with an opened spoon; channel well on paper towels.

2.   Preheat broiler to 450°. Spot cauliflower on a lubed wire rack in a

15x10x1-in. heating dish. Prepare on a lower broiler rack until dim brilliant, 39 minutes.

3.   In the meantime, place almonds, bread morsels, tomatoes, cooked peppers, parsley, garlic, paprika, salt, and pepper in a nourishment processor; beat until finely cleaved. Include remaining sherry; process until mixed. Keep preparing while step by step including remaining oil in a constant flow. Present with cauliflower.

Spicy Grilled Broccoli

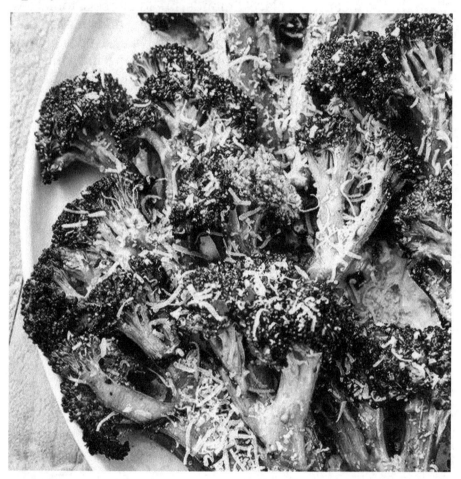

Total Time

Prep: 20 min. + standing Grill: 10 min.

Makes

6 servings

Ingredients:

- 2 packs broccoli

MARINADE:

1/2 cup olive oil

- 1/4 cup juice vinegar

- 1 teaspoon onion powder

- 1 teaspoon garlic powder

- 1 teaspoon smoked paprika

- 1/2 teaspoon salt

- 1/2 teaspoon squashed red pepper pieces 1/4 teaspoon pepper

Direction:

1.   Cut every broccoli pack into 6 pieces. In a 6-qt. stockpot, place a steamer container more than 1 in. of water. Spot broccoli in bushel. Heat water to the point of boiling. Decrease warmth to keep up a stew; steam, secured, 4-6 minutes or until fresh delicate.

2.   In an enormous bowl, whisk marinade fixings until mixed. Include broccoli; delicately hurl to cover. Let stand, secured, 15 minutes.

3.   Channel broccoli, saving marinade. Flame broil broccoli, secured, over medium warmth or cook 4 in. from heat 6-8 minutes or until

broccoli is delicate, turning once. Whenever wanted, present withheld marinade.

CPSIA information can be obtained
at www.ICGtesting.com
Printed in the USA
BVHW090910260421
605849BV00002B/125

9 781802 690712